Nursing the Nurse

Printed in the United States of America

First Printing, January 2001
ISBN 1-56533-040-4

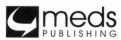

Suite 260
4000 Blackburn Lane
Burtonsville, MD 20866
301-476-9666
www.medspub.com

Nursing
the Nurse

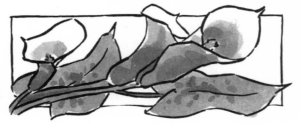

Affirmations

Gail Staudt, MSN, RN, CS

*Dedicated in loving memory of my Mother,
whose words of wisdom set the foundation
for my thought processes in life.*

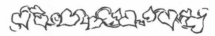

Foreword

These affirmations are a tribute to all of my colleagues who may leave work at the end of the shift tired and exhausted. It is written for those who may have been so busy that they never got their break or may not have had time for lunch; who may have learned that many of us have achieved the bladder training of a camel and the tolerance of a saint. The words within are meant to help you to put things in perspective when the world is a whirlwind around you and people expect you to remain strong and durable. I hope that these thoughts will provide some introspection, validation, and encouragement when no one else is around to tell you how important you are to the human spirit.

It has been said that people come into and out of our lives for a reason and that is for us to learn. The path that I have followed to self awareness and personal growth has been paved by many of my colleagues. I am so thankful to them for being part of the guidance that God has provided to me. Their support and friendship have been my life lessons. My "nurse-teachers" are too numerous to mention, but special recognition must be given to some who have been my support at significant times of transition. Among them are: Doris Maurer, Carolyn Thomas, Karen Talerico, Ilene Prokop, Janet Sipple, Carol Sorrentino, Toni Bereskie, Judy Gill, Susan York, Wanda Mohr, Linda Goldberg, Emma Rahn, Gloria Miller, Kim Johnston, Joanne Gillis-Donovan, Cheryl Knabb, Freida Outlaw, Debbie Levengood, Delores Yundt, Sharry Carrigan, Leanne Zeiber, Bert Stichter, and all of those others who have crossed my path and offered themselves to me.

May this book provide you with some of those lessons that these people have taught me.

—Gail Staudt
October 1999

*The Language of Flowers

Calla Lily... balance
Rose Geranium... preference
Ivy... friendship
Heliotrope... devotion
Pansy... thoughts

*from *Home Remedies for Man and Beast*
A Complete Manual of Domestic Information.
by Prof. B. G. Jefferis, M. D., Ph. D.
1892

Contents

Create your life the way you want it to be.

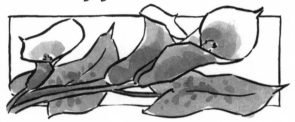

CALLA LILY • BALANCE

1 No one can be as hard on us as we are on ourselves. Many of us learned that if we make a mistake it is a character flaw. By necessity, the nursing profession demands perfection, as well. But, life is not perfect! We all have made mistakes along the way. So often, though, we keep the label that we have put on ourselves from the past. We then apply it to the event at hand as though it is an extension of our faulty self. We say things like—"But, I have always been like this," or "You don't understand me—I have a bad running record," or "How could I have been so stupid?" Our past doesn't have to be a permanent condition. Learn from it. Take it as a life lesson to be learned. Deal with the issue of today and let go of it. Get rid of the self-label. Even corporations change logos from time to time.

Today is the day that I will change my logo. My new logo will be a positive one.

Be gentle with yourself.

2 We give our energy to people all day long. As caregivers we are expected to be able to do that. The problem is that we often forget to take care of ourselves after the workday is over. After putting so much out, we need to take some energy in. "Me" time is important. It can take the form of a special day off, or simple things such as bubble baths or ordering a pizza instead of cooking dinner. What is important is to re-fuel. Even our cars run out of gas if we don't refill the tank.

Taking time to relax will help me. It is not a selfish thing to do, but rather, is a self-caring thing.

Feel your feelings.

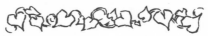

3 To be "professional" usually means that we don't show our real feelings. Over time we can build resentment, anger, and other negative attitudes if we don't release our frustrations. Anger and frustration are negative energy. It is okay to vent in an appropriate way, that is, a way that doesn't harm someone else or yourself. The trick is to find the one that works for you. Some of my clients have found relief in a variety of ways. Some unique ones include slamming phone books on the floor, punching a pillow or punching bag, journaling, or throwing Playdough against a wall. A really creative "Open-Heart" nurse that I know went to a flea market, bought a cheap set of dishes, and threw them, one at a time, at a tree. She felt better afterwards. The worst part was the cleanup.

It is important that I find a helpful way to vent my feelings without harming others or myself. Today is the day that I will find that way.

*Even when it feels
personal, it may not be.*

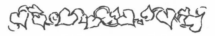

4 I have noticed a tendency for nurses to get angry when they feel vulnerable. We may not realize it at the time, but we usually seem to feel anger when we are out of control of a situation. It has been a difficult thing to learn, but I now try to ask myself the following question when I feel angry: "What is going on with me in this situation?" So often the answer has very little to do with the person who is "making me angry." It doesn't seem to matter whether that person is a patient, physician, nurse-colleague, or a personal relationship. I have found that I am responding to the situation based on past experience and my buttons are being pushed. It helps to remember that no one can push our buttons unless we have them to push.

If I begin to feel impatient or angry, I will try to take some time to look at what is going on with me before I blame the other person.

Decide what you believe in and then decide what you want to do about it.

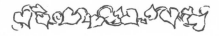

5 True peace and serenity come from within. It may take some doing to find it. Sometimes it takes a fair amount of effort to sift through the accumulated hurt and other feelings that may be blocking our ability to truly feel good. Add to that the fact that we are supposed to look strong all of the time, and it is an almost impossible task. I admire those nurses with whom I have worked in my practice along the way. Their ability to seek some assistance to sort through their "stuff" is a sign of strength. To me, they are the strong ones. It is a sad thing to know that so many nurses may not have the courage at the moment to deal with the pain that they carry. I consider it a privilege to work with my clients. It is truly a joy to watch them grow.

Growth is like surgery.
We often need to face the pain
of the experience in order to start
to heal. Today I will decide those
things that I believe in for myself
and then answer the question
of what I want to do about
that belief.

Selfcare is not selfish.

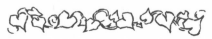

6 Spirituality is an interesting word. Many see the word defined as one that connotes a religious belief. But, in fact, the spirit encompasses more than that. Those who practice within a holistic nursing framework understand that optimal health occurs when not only the physical symptoms are addressed, but when the emotional and spiritual self are addressed, as well. Most nurses are in touch with that at some level. We do things like spend time talking to a distraught patient, talking about patient's feelings, or offering a form of therapeutic touch (holding a hand, massaging, etc.). So many of us are holistic nurses and are addressing the spirituality needs of our patients without even realizing it. But, in order to nurture our patient's spirituality, we need to nurture our own. I guess we are back to the need for balance in life again!

Today I will do something to
promote my own inner peace.
By doing so, I will be able to
provide better care to my patients.

Tears heal.

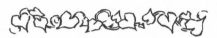

7 Crying can be very cathartic. There is evidence that speaks to the biochemical release of toxins when we are upset and can have a good cry. But, it isn't that simple for nurses. We are accustomed to "being professional," especially in crisis. How effective would we be if we became emotional during an emergency? In fact, we have become conditioned to suppress any emotion during a crisis. So conditioned that I have talked to nurses who describe the inability to cry at all. They explain that there is the feeling that they may need to cry, they may even well up with tears, but it "just doesn't come." The price that is paid is to have some type of physical problem such as headaches, back pain, eating disorders, or the like. Or, they have episodes of panic attack-type feelings. Such suppressed emotional pain is a heavy load to carry. There is another way to feel. We may need a therapist to coach us through the process.

I need to feel my feelings in order to move forward. I will try to acknowledge my feelings rather than "stuff" them.

Don't panic,
there is <u>always</u> a choice.

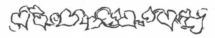

8 Once, as a nurse manager of an ICU, I facilitated a staff meeting where the conversation turned towards the placement of necessary emergency equipment at the patients' bedsides. It was amazing to me that we could not get a consensus opinion of what was needed at each patient's unit. Here we were, eight nurses who make instantaneous life and death decisions on a daily basis, and we couldn't problem-solve such a simple question. After pondering the situation, I wondered if our struggle had something to do with each of us having a different perception about what the perfect answer would be. I suspect this to be the case. It really held up progressing to the next issue. But, how does one conduct a democratic process in such an instance? I guess that on some occasions it would be helpful to find the gray areas instead of being so black and white about our options.

I will try to view as many options as I can when faced with a situation. There are always choices. Thinking in extremes does not give us the whole picture.

Decelerate!

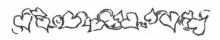

9 So many nurses have difficulty sleeping. The common story goes something like this: the nurse will go to bed, and due to exhaustion, will fall asleep. Several hours later, the eyes pop open and the person feels wide-awake. After pacing the hall, fatigue sets in and the person may be able to go back to sleep. Sure enough, the alarm goes off shortly thereafter, and it is time to go to work. Having been deprived of a good, deep, REM sleep, the individual is fatigued before the day even begins. Now, I know that none of us can walk down a unit hallway and look straight ahead. We scan the area as we go, looking in each patient room as we pass. We are scanning for abnormalities that may need to be addressed. It continues as a reflex no matter where we are. This conditioned behavior involves a level of hyper-vigilance. If we don't do something to tell our brain that it is time to rest, we will continue to be hyper-vigilant as we fall asleep. Since we are not using up the adrenaline that we are producing, it will catch up to us after several hours, and we will awaken. It is so much easier to take ten minutes before bed to deliver a calming message to our brain. Looking at a magazine, reading a book, taking a warm bath, or having a cup of warm milk may help the process. Stress management can take so little time.

Taking a few moments
to care for myself before sleep will
help me to be more rested.

Each day contains gifts.

ROSE GERANIUM • PREFERENCE

10 It's difficult for some of us to leave our own families and go to work on a holiday. It starts with the schedule going up, which may bother us until the day arrives and we get to work. Actually, if we are willing to be honest, the thought of working on a holiday is sometimes worse than the actual day itself. If we think about the positives of working on a holiday, it may not be as upsetting. Positives?? Well, we get to go home after our shift—our patients don't. Also, we can enjoy the lack of administrative activity that occurs on a holiday. I have always enjoyed the fact that holiday work was purely about giving good patient care. The whole focus is on giving the care on a day when the managerial tedium is put on the back burner. In addition, the holiday pay check can be helpful— I always give myself an extra treat with the extra income. Yep, the positives!

I will look for the good parts of today and celebrate them.

In order to grow,
we need to reach out
beyond ourselves.

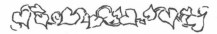

11 For some of us, holidays are a lonely time and we seek out the ability to work instead of dealing with the issues in our personal lives. While our co-workers may appreciate the chance to have off, it is important for us to have some time off as well. While working on a holiday may provide us with a reason not to deal with our personal "stuff," we usually build anger about this over time. Using the work schedule to hide from our own personal issues will not work. After the shift, the issues are still there. Working on a holiday will only be a temporary solution. Spending time with those who are willing to nurture you is much more helpful. Plan ahead for such a time. Let your friends know you need something to do. It can be a validating feeling to have an invitation—even if it isn't from whom you are seeking it. Sometimes we look for others to give what they just don't have to give, while we miss out on those who are willing to give. When we hide at work, we are non-verbally asking our patients to take care of us instead of vice versa.

I will plan ahead to make the next holiday the best that I can make it. I will reach out to others if I need someone to be with.

Ask for what you need.

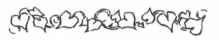

12 Some holidays are more special than others. For some it may be Christmas, for others Kwanzaa or Hanukkah. Getting our favorite holiday off may not be an option. We may be expected to take our turn with our peers. But, we may be able to trade with someone else or make another arrangement. It is important to remember that the first concern to a nurse manager is to have enough staff for patient care. Our needs may be met along with that concern. Life always provides options. It is up to us to find them. We are more apt to get our needs met if we ask our manager for assistance in identifying those options rather than pressuring him/her to fix it for us. Be part of the solution instead of part of the problem.

*I will take responsibility for
my needs, and ask for assistance
to get my needs met.*

Be loved.

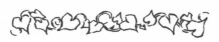

13 Sometime we may feel anger towards our patients when we must work on a holiday. We may feel that it is because of them that we are required to be on duty. Unfortunately, illness and need have no respect for holidays. I have already seen nurses miss out on the signs of appreciation that are given by patients and family members on holidays. Look for these. It certainly helps and reminds us of the reasons why we are caregivers in the first place.

Holidays are times of joy.
I will be aware of those joys that
will pass my way today.

Lighten up.

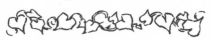

14 So many of us are nurses because we learned to take care of others within our families. The problem is that when we take the role of the "strong one," we are expected to always be that. We usually have a full day of nursing, go home, and nurse some more. Unfortunately, there are times when we need support, as well. And, during those times, we may be reluctant to ask for it. Or, in some instances, those around us may not be able to give it. Sometimes, the best support comes from unlikely friendships. Look around you for those who don't have as high an expectation of you and who may reach back when you reach out. You may be pleasantly surprised!

Trying to make someone do what he/she is not able to do is frustrating to everyone concerned. I will look for those who are available to me instead of expecting it from someone who is not able to do it.

In a difficult situation ask yourself, "What part am I playing in this?"

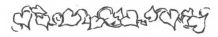

15 Reaching out can be difficult. When we have been expected to be able to handle situations of all sorts on a regular basis, we may develop the "Super-person" syndrome. That is, needing to be needed, and therefore, being all things to all people. Only when we have accumulated a pile of disappointments and stresses, do we look for support. Usually by then, we are so angry because no one has helped us up to that point. Maybe a better way is to take care of matters along the way before they get to the point of crisis. Or—is it that we are choosing to be all things to all people? If so, maybe we are creating our own situations while blaming others. Learning to care for yourself while caring for others may be helpful.

It may be helpful to be aware of the part that I play in my life situations. By focusing on myself, I may not be as ready to blame others.

Take your time.

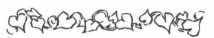

16 It is amazing to me how many of us feel responsible for the personal struggles of those around us. There is a danger when we "need to be needed." The problem is that often our motivation has more to do with our need to feel good about ourselves than it does about helping others. Some people call it "Helper's High." We tend to use the nursing process by thinking that if we can identify the problem and offer an opinion, we can "fix" it. Unfortunately, we aren't that powerful. It takes some of us quite awhile to figure that out. We usually come to realize it when we are met with resistance or we don't see the result that we wanted. A healthier approach is to identify options for others and to allow them to choose the one that is effective for them. This may take time and may involve some choices that don't necessarily work until he/she sorts it out. Things just may not work out on our schedule—but that doesn't mean that eventually it may not work out.

Things may not happen on my schedule. If I want to help others, I need to allow them the space that they may need to make their own decisions.

*Life cannot unravel
when we tie knots in it.*

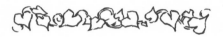

17 So many of us have never come to realize that we can't be in control of everything in life. We may get ourselves into trouble trying to control everyone and everything around us. What a stressful set of circumstances we create for ourselves, and we don't even know that we are doing it. The problem is that what we do well at work—taking control—can convert to a real social problem in our personal lives. It is important to learn how to "let go" of situations, even when it means that someone we love may need to struggle through their own learning process. The fact is that if we continuously rescue people from situations, they never learn to do it for themselves. I guess that means we may be getting in the way of their healing when we think that we are promoting it. Hmm, interesting!

Letting go does not mean abandoning others. Rather it is a way to allow others to find their own way. That can be a loving thing to do.

Accept support.

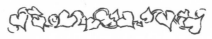

18 I have had conversations with nurses who tell me that they are unable to cry, even though it would make them feel better. A common concern is a fear of the loss of control. That is, that if he/she allows him/herself to cry, he/she may lose control to the point that he/she may not be able to regain it. I would like to say this: It may feel that way, but it just won't happen. When we are so accustomed to being so in control, it is a frightening thing to consider another option. But, relief is like surgery—we need to feel pain, in order to feel better. Healing will happen if we allow ourselves to feel. I suggest that you have some type of help to do this. Get support in order to process it away. After all, we would never do our own surgery!

I do not have to do anything alone. I can have help on my journey.

Create joy.

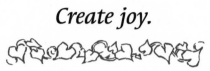

19 I remember the first day of grad school. My professor entered the classroom and, before saying hello, asked how many of us were the first-born in our family or were asked to act as the first-born. All but two of the fifteen or so students raised their hand. As she scanned the room, she zeroed in on those without their hand raised and replied, "You just don't realize it yet." As we all know, the usual role of the first-born is to be the role model, protector, and caregiver for our younger siblings. What great preparation for the future! We were to understand later that the majority of us entered nursing in order to do what we already learned to do along the way. That is, to take care of others, frequently at our own expense. It is no wonder we have burnout occurring!

I will balance my life by doing some special things for myself, especially when I am doing a lot of caring of others.

Feelings aren't good or bad,
they just are.

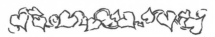

20 Another's anger is always a difficult thing to manage. I have found that many of us respond to what other people think. If it is a negative opinion, we may feel that we must do something about it, even though deep down we may feel that the argument is not logical. It is important to know that, just because someone has an opinion, it doesn't mean that they are correct. Take time to ask yourself the question, "Does what is being said belong to me?" You may find that it doesn't. Remember the defense mechanism of projection that we were taught in Psych classes. In case you don't remember, it is when someone projects his/her feelings onto another. Keep it in mind. It is okay to tell someone that what they are saying does not belong to you or that they have a right to an opinion, but that isn't how you see it.

I will trust my opinion about myself. While it is worthwhile to consider another's viewpoint, I am not obligated to accept it.

Peace and serenity
come from within.

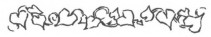

21 Caring does not mean "fixing." It is difficult to sort out these two concepts. The determining factor is whether or not another involved individual wants our assistance in a given situation. Our nursing work requires us to assess events and to provide a therapeutic intervention. But, in our personal lives, there are times when it is more beneficial to allow someone to find their own way. I have found these to be very challenging times. The Serenity Prayer has been helpful.

"God grant me the serenity to accept the things I cannot change; the courage to change the things I can; and the wisdom to know the difference." I will attempt to define what is changeable and what is not.

*Seek common ground
with others.*

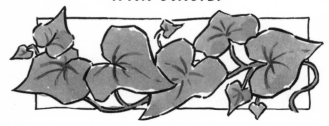

IVY • FRIENDSHIP

22 A rule of thumb is that organizations will do what they think that they need to do in order to survive. In today's healthcare industry there are a lot of changes made by the hierarchy. Administrative decisions are not personal, even though they may often feel that way. The difficult thing is that we, as nurses, are praised for our reactivity at work when it impacts patient care, but that very same response, which earns us nursing recognition and awards, is viewed as negative when we react to organizational issues. It is a hard thing to sort out, but it is crucial to our ability to cope within organizations that we learn the art of negotiation. That means learning to speak the language of the executive. Administrators are more apt to understand issues if they are expressed in terms that they comprehend. Now more than ever, communication skills are crucial.

When I can negotiate, I resolve problems to everyone's benefit. In doing so, I need to actively listen to another's point of view as well as express mine in a logical way.

Scan your horizons.

23 We need to read every newspaper, magazine, and journal and listen to every news story with a key question in mind— "How might this impact my practice?" It is ironic how we may see new technologies and not think about how that very procedure or new piece of equipment may cause a decrease in personnel requirements. There is a rule of business—"Look for the unlikely competitor." The postal service has been impacted by fax machines and email. Where is the unlikely competition for your position?

Helpful information is everywhere. I will pay attention to all of those hints that may pass my way today.

Share yourself with others.

24 We have often been shy about telling people why we, as nurses, are important to patient care. We feel that we are bragging. The price that we pay is that very few people really know what a nurse does. Describing our roles and role function is crucial. If we don't explain to others our vast array of skills, how will they know? Instead of feeling as though you are "bragging," view it as "educating" others. If we don't tell others what we are capable of, how will they know?

Educating others about my nursing role will help them to be aware of their resources for health and wellness.

You are important.

25 Nurses are truly special. My personal opinion, biased of course, is that our uniqueness lies in our ability to bridge the physiological with the psychosocial aspects of illness and wellness. Some call it a holistic approach. Unfortunately, it is so innate in us that we don't even realize the specialness of it. This focus on health is so very important to our ability to facilitate healing. To care for the emotional well-being of another while also concurrently caring for the physical issues is an incredible talent. Yes, we are truly special.

*I am special for the work that I do
and the person that I am.
I will keep that in mind as I go
through my day today.*

Proactivity
outweighs reactivity.

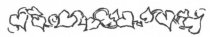

26 It has been said that to try to get nurses to work together is to try to herd cats. This philosophy was said in a political sense. We pay a price when we are not able to support each other within our profession. The biggest consequence is that we have really struggled to define our own practice in an evolving healthcare climate. We need to become more aware of the political and practice issues that are occurring as the climate changes around us. If we don't become part of the process, others will control our practice as nurses. Our tendency when this does happen is for us to take on a victim role. "They are doing this to us." It is vital that we learn to be proactive by supporting our professional organizations. It is too late when someone has assumed our roles or has passed a law to undermine our practice. In today's world we are vulnerable to individuals who follow a "divide and conquer" strategy.

I am part of a very special profession. I will support my peers by mentoring, offering assistance, and getting involved. And, I will accept support when it is offered.

Think excellence
but strive for the best
that you can do.

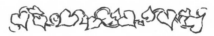

27 It makes me sad when I hear nurses say, if they had it to do all over again, they would not be nurses. I can't help but feel that this is said by someone who has not looked at all the opportunities that the profession has to offer. It is uttered by those who are drained, and not able to nurture themselves, in the midst of their caregiving. I have found the profession to offer a gamut of opportunities to us. My background includes Critical Care nursing, Nephrology/Hemodialysis nursing, teaching, psychiatric advanced practice, legal nurse consulting, expert witnessing, and management. Yet, there are so many areas that I haven't tried. Some of us hold conversations by complaining. Maybe, when someone says that he/she would not be a nurse again, they are just holding a conversation.

To complain is to spend time doing something that does not resolve the problem. I will look for ways to grow by seizing opportunities when they present themselves. Even small changes such as membership on a committee may offer new insight.

If you don't speak up,
no one will know.

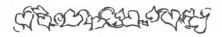

28 We eat our young. There are all kinds of philosophies about why we have difficulty teaching and supporting the new nurse. It may go back to the expectations that we have towards ourselves and others. Or, it might be that we are not happy with life, in general. Most of us are impatient to see results. I call it the "Give 'em Lasix, watch them void" mentality. Growth is a process. Educators call it a learning curve. In other words, learning takes time. What I know is that if we don't look at this issue, be supportive preceptors, and address the issue on an individual basis, we are not doing anything to further our profession. If we don't support our profession and those in it, do we have the right to complain about it?

I have a lot to offer to those with whom I work. Those around me will not be helped by my life experience unless I share it with them. I will try to take the time to educate my co-workers.

Play fair.

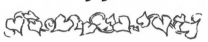

29 There is a theory that speaks to Horizontal Violence existing in our profession. The concept that the theory describes is that nurses reflect a similar phenomenon common to prisoners of war. The dynamic issue is the behaviors that occur when we feel somewhat powerless in our circumstances and do not feel safe to express our concerns to those in authority. The end result is that we take our frustrations out on each other. I have noticed this repeatedly amongst our peers. It takes the form of reporting each other, of not supporting each other's efforts, of talking in a negative fashion about each other, and similar behaviors. I hope that we catch on to this some day. It would make our profession a whole lot stronger if we could work together. Maybe it can start with each one of us.

I will do my best to support my peers and to approach misunderstandings in a way that each of us may be able to express a view and have it respected by the other side.

Take "me" time.

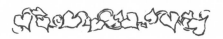

30 I have been part of several conversations with my peers that discussed the meaning of the word "collaboration." Some nurses view collaboration as the ability to work in a compatible fashion with other disciplines in healthcare. But, when one looks at the nursing role being performed in some of those instances, one sees a nursing function of extending another's practice rather than expanding the nursing role. This is an important thing to work out in our profession. It makes a difference in terms of defining the way we can practice, and also who defines our practice—whether an Advanced Practice nurse should be mandated to be supervised or not or whether we are able to practice in an autonomous fashion. Any way you look at it, we need to be part of the conversation in order to facilitate the evolution of the nursing role. None of us is absolved from this duty. More importantly, our patients deserve for us to be the most skilled, competent and caring nurses that we can be. We cannot fulfill those requirements unless we are clear about our practice standards. We are not powerless in this regard, but we need to learn to speak up.

I will care for my clients by caring for myself and by taking an active part in defining nursing practice.

Share your wealth.

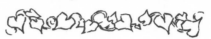

31 I had a public relations friend who said that what she noticed about us was that nurses traveled in packs. At first I laughed, but then I became more attentive to why she said that. The fact is that I noticed us doing just that. When I looked around the hospital cafeteria or when I went to a conference, there we were—glued at the hip. I suppose that it shouldn't be surprising. There is a certain camaraderie that is developed when we can identify with each other's situations and concerns. But, it might broaden our horizons if we stretched beyond the line of nursing and got to know other co-workers a bit better.

*I will make an attempt
to improve my contact with
members of other disciplines.
Doing so will be an educational
experience for each side.*

Expect respect.

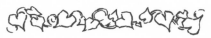

32 What do you do if you are the subject of a doctor's anger? I have seen nurses respond in a variety of ways. Of special concern is the nurse who appears submissive and victimized. But, the nurse who becomes angry and defends him/herself in a loud fashion is just as disconcerting. The fact is that there is no problem resolution in either circumstance. This means that the issue spurns emotions that will be unfinished and just add fuel to the next round that is apt to happen. It is important to set limits about the anger of another. When they are fired up is not the time to continue the conversation. It has always worked for me to use the quietest tone of voice that I can muster and offer to talk to them later when they are able to help to solve the problem. I then sever myself from the conversation until things defuse. It takes practice, but I have found that, after a few times of doing this, I was no longer the target during future events.

We are all professionals in our own right. Being reactive to another's abusive behavior is non-productive. I can set limits on those behaviors that are acceptable to me.

A caring touch
speaks louder than words.

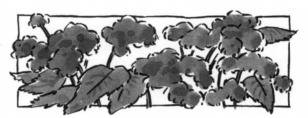

HELIOTROPE • DEVOTION

33 I believe that patients go through the stages of the grieving process as they experience the loss of health. Just the label of a diagnosis can initiate the event. That includes denial of the situation, bargaining, anger, and depression. Sometimes, as nurses, the only patients that we like are the ones who have accepted their disease and follow all of our directions. If we can remember that part of our job is to help them get from denial to the stage of acceptance, it makes it a bit easier. If we can't, the therapeutic relationship turns into a power struggle. Any way you look at it, we nurses are in control of the situation. It's up to us to set the pace.

All behavior has meaning.
If I can meet my patients where
they are, I will be more likely
to promote healing.

Take time
to act your shoe size.

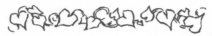

34 We forget that our usual work environment is a negative one. On a daily basis, we are dealing with illness, depression, people's troubles, and death and dying. To us, these events can feel commonplace and our perception of the normal world can become distorted. The fact of the matter is that the majority of the world is not as unhealthy and struggling. It is so important to re-center ourselves after a day of work. I might suggest some of the things that have worked for me. I stay away from the news for awhile, play soft music in my car, choose funny movies to see, and I have never seen any of the hospital-based TV shows, on purpose. And, I stay away from soap operas, as well. The bottom line is that our own wellness depends on balance. If we are in a negative environment for any period of time, we need to seek positive energy in order to regain balance.

I will begin to surround myself with leisure-time activities and people who will help me to gain positive energy and to regain some balance in my life.

My schedule
may not be everyone else's.

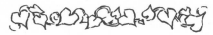

35 Have you ever asked yourself why you became a nurse? Many of us say that it is because we want to "take care of people." Often this translates into "fixing" people. The difference in definitions is reflected in how we deliver care and the expectations that we place on our patients to follow our instructions. Or, to second-guess ourselves if the patient does not improve, often thinking that we may have missed something. This is an important concept since it determines the ability for us to accommodate a therapeutic relationship or to feel job satisfaction. The end result is that we tend to blame another, or ourselves, when someone does not improve, or to take credit for someone getting better. In any event, the process has us as the focus instead of the patient.

Healing is a process,
not an event that happens.
Today I will focus on the needs
of my patients and respect
their choices.

Focus on you.

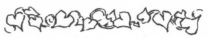

36 Have you ever watched one nurse give report to another nurse? So much can be told by watching this exchange. Issues of camaraderie and professionalism become apparent. Is there patience regarding the reporting nurse's style of delivery? Do issues that occur between shifts become apparent? Is the oncoming nurse paying attention to what is said? We tend to take our frustrations out on each other at times. Perhaps it would help to look at the real issue at hand. Could it be fatigue, personal issues, worry, or anger over something totally unrelated? Dealing with the real issue can help our relationships and improve communication, as well. A lot also has to do with how we tell a story. Some of us get into a lot of detail; some of us are much more succinct. Nurses in fast-paced areas such as ERs and ICUs tend to be the latter, more compact and more left-brained. Unfortunately, while this is helpful to their decision-making, those not as linear-thinking may interpret it as rude. It really is the way that they process information.

Doing things differently than I do does not mean that it is being done incorrectly. If I can learn not to judge others around me, I may find that my relationships will improve. I can make a difference in my own small way.

Diversify.

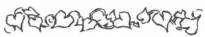

37 Are you one of those nurses who can't start your shift until you rearrange the work area? Being organized is a good thing, unless it is a compulsive habit. If this whole concept brings a smile to your face, you are probably one of " them." The main problem has more to do with the anger that comes with this behavior. The anger is usually directed at the preceding nurse who didn't leave the world in the order that we consider perfect. And so, the question becomes: "Is the actual issue a disheveled room/work area, or is it that your anxiety level is up because your co-worker does not do things exactly the way you do?" I have found this to be a particular problem in areas where quantities of equipment are necessary at the patient's bedside. There is more than one way to do most things. This is a hard thing to remember and even to understand in an environment of linear items such as clinical pathways and forms of all sorts. The problem is, if we are too rigid, the anger accompanying it will take its toll on us. Is it really worth it?

Getting my work area in the order that I want it may not necessarily mean that someone else's version of the arrangement may have been wrong.

Take your time.

38 We have a unique way of thinking known as the nursing process. It is so ingrained in us that we don't know that others may not think as systematically as we do. It is second nature for us to look at almost any situation and assess it, by finding a meaning to what we see, deciding what to do about it, and then looking for a result that is more effective than what we started out with. Now, while this method makes us extremely competent and useful in the clinical setting, in our personal life, it can set us up to be considered over-analytical by our non-nursing counterparts. It is a tendency that we have, and it is good self-awareness, to consider this as a factor in any conflicts. It is a gift, as well, valued by many of our professional colleagues—and of definite worth to our patients.

Being analytical is not a character flaw. However, I will be careful not to expect immediate results.

Know that you did your best.

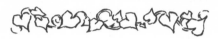

39 I doubt that there is a nurse who is reading this who hasn't seen someone die or has witnessed the process of dying at one point in his/her career. Years later, there are those that I still remember. It was especially difficult since, starting at the age of twenty-one, I worked in an Intensive Care Unit in the same town in which I grew up. As result, I saw people that I knew as a child go through the end-of-life process. I thought that I handled it relatively well, and I did, but in retrospect, I think that these experiences had more impact on me than I originally thought.

I will be gentle with myself
and acknowledge my feelings
when I lose a patient.
If necessary, I will seek assistance
from another.

As I give, so can I receive.

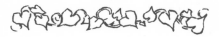

40 There was a time when I struggled with the fact that children die. Somehow, I could accept an adult's death by rationalizing that he or she had lived a particular length of time. But, I had difficulty making sense of a child's death. Then, I went to graduate school. One of my professors made a comment one day that really struck home. "People come in and out of our lives for a reason," she said, "and that is for us to learn." What a profound statement! Could it be, perhaps, that a child's purpose is to be here to deliver a lesson, to bring people closer, or to get people in touch with what is important in life?

I will reflect on what my patients are teaching me as they go through their own life processes.

Learn from others.

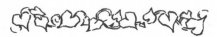

41 The power of the human spirit is an incredible thing. As we have cared for patients, so many of us have seen the person who has given up and dies for no obvious emergent reason. Or, the patient who announces his death, which then occurs as predicted. Or, the patient in critical condition who is, for all intents and purposes, brain dead and/or ventilator-dependent, and who stays alive until that family member arrives from out-of-town and then passes in a very short period of time. Many of us have gained a healthy respect for the apparent control of the mind-body connection and the power we hold over our own demise.

I will listen to what my patients are telling me so that I may be aware of their needs.

Change is an opportunity for opportunities.

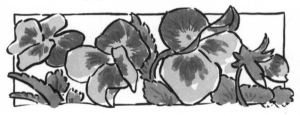

PANSY • THOUGHTS

42 Change is constant. It is helpful to look for those "red flags" that will indicate what might be happening. For example, articles regarding new patient care delivery systems, management styles, or new expressions that are being used more frequently may be introductions of things to come. "Red flags" are not meant to cause us panic, but are helpful to pre-warn us of things to come. They may be quite helpful to us so that we can figure out our options should change occur. If you see "red flags," don't panic—just start to develop a plan B.

Change is a process, not an event.
I will be aware of the process
and take care of myself within it.

If it's uncomfortable,
get rid of it.

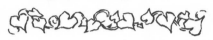

43 Coping with stress can be a really difficult thing to do. We all do something to cope. Some of us drink, gamble, exercise, eat, or don't eat, etc., etc. Nurses seem to lean toward socially acceptable things in excess. A big one is shopping. A nurse that I know had a very difficult day. She came home and looked at her mail. There she found a popular catalogue. She went through it, picked out her items, and placed her phone order for $800. The next day she signed up for three extra shifts in order to pay for her purchases. What she didn't realize was that she was putting herself back into the very situation that caused her stress in the first place. While shopping is a benign event unto itself, anything can get us into trouble when done in excess.

Stress is a part of life. However, if I find that I have a need to use my chosen coping skill in excess, I will look to see what is causing me so much anxiety and do something about it.

Create your own destiny.

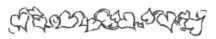

44 Another nurse that I know told me how she felt when she went shopping. She had filed for bankruptcy and was trying to figure out how not to get into credit card trouble again. With a glazed look in her eyes, she told me that, when she entered a store, everything seemed to be stacked in neat piles and in order. She talked about how nice it felt to be in such an orderly environment. She concluded that buying something was her effort to take a piece of that orderliness home with her. Unfortunately, it didn't work since the adrenaline surge only lasted for a few moments at the time of the sale. Research has shown that there is a feeling of physiologically-based euphoria surrounding these events. But, it doesn't get the job done. Looking outside of ourselves is not the right place to find a sense of peace.

According to the Dalai Lama, we are all seeking a higher level of happiness. This is not something that can be purchased, ingested or inhaled. Looking for peace starts with looking for the gaps in our own selves and starting to fill them. Today I will start the search.

*Refuel your soul
before you run out of gas.*

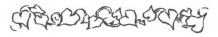

45 Mental Health days are about balance. We need a day off when we have given so much to everyone for so long that, when we wake up in the morning, we just don't have it to give. We have run out of energy. It is amazing how nurses describe that it isn't only the day off, but the feeling of having gotten away with something that is helpful. But, there are also feelings of guilt, as well. This will add to the stress, in the long term. A better way is to nurture ourselves as we go, instead of needing time off in one burst of a day.

Today I will begin a new daily habit. I will identify two positive things that occurred in my life today and I will take ten minutes before going to bed to do some quiet activity that will nurture me.

The pains of life
are often growing pains.

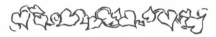

46 I have come across an old saying, "If our eyes don't cry, our organs will." Necessary emotional release is vital to well-being. I suggest that, if you relate to this dilemma, you might want to find someone to talk to in order to deal with it. Many, many years ago, I thought an epigastric knot was a normal feeling to have on a daily basis. What a relief to know that I don't have to carry that feeling with me. In fact, if I feel any indications of it, I immediately start to look at what is going on in my life to produce tension. It is such a relief to find another way.

The pain that I sometimes feel is growing pain. I will find a way to release my pain so that it does not hold so much power over me.

Make a decision,
then move on.

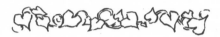

47 So many of us have extremely high expectations of ourselves. I have repeatedly observed this, but it became very obvious during the years that I taught at a university. The program was an RN to BSN program where most of the students were non-traditional, seasoned nurses. It was a joy to teach those who had so much life experience to share. The classes were quite interesting and the students had so much to do with that. They had so many life stories to tell. But, the biggest challenge was the issue of how to evaluate student performance. One of the common issues was the grading system. So many nurses would be upset if they didn't get an "A" grade. A "B" was often treated as a personal failing grade. As a professor, it felt as though, instead of starting the course with a goal of earning the "A," some students seemed to assume that they deserved an "A" unless proven otherwise. Perfectionism can get really frustrating for all concerned.

Striving to do things well is a positive thing. However, if I am not perfect, that doesn't mean I've failed.

Breathe!

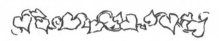

48 Have you ever noticed all the stimuli that you are subject to while at work? So many sounds to acknowledge, process, and react to—monitors alarming, people talking, patients calling, pumps beeping, ventilators buzzing, pagers beeping, cell phones ringing, and on and on. It is amazing how much sensory overload nurses can handle. If we want to be balanced, it is crucial to offset the noise with some quiet time. It can be done quickly—even at work. If you are feeling overstimulated, try "one-nostril breathing." Close your mouth and, by using your fingers to press your nostrils, breathe in one nostril and then close that nostril and breathe out the other. Repeat this process taking as slow and deep breaths as possible three times. Then alternate to the opposite side for three deep breaths. You should now feel a bit calmer. What you have done is to reduce your air passages by one-half causing you to take in less room air and to exhale less carbon dioxide. The end result is the retention of carbon dioxide, which has a natural sedative effect. And, it only took six breaths!

Practicing a coping technique is best done prior to the crisis. I will try a new strategy before I need it.

Enjoy life's gifts.

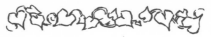

49 I think it's the funniest thing when, at a party or other social event, the nurses at the occasion can find each other. Even though they may have never met, they quickly form a huddle and proceed to compare notes regarding their jobs. I might mention that it usually isn't a brief exchange, either. Now, while this is occurring, other occupational groups don't seem to be gathered. So, how come nurses single themselves out? It might be that we have a very difficult time separating our work life from our personal life. Or is it that we don't feel as secure among people outside the healthcare arena? Perhaps, is it that we interact with each other because we speak the same language? Perhaps, there is another reason. Whatever the reason, when we do this, nurses miss an opportunity to know others and to get away from the job for a period of time.

I will keep social time as social time. If my work is all I have to talk about, I will take that as a sign that I need to seek more leisure-time activity.

Life's too short to waste.

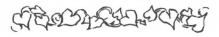

50 I am a single woman; a Catholic; a daughter; an educator; a lecturer; an older sister; a therapist; a writer; a business woman; a niece; a clothes horse; a jewelry collector; an aunt; a walker; an exerciser [when time permits]; an entrepreneur; a traveler; a Scrabble player; a friend; an okay cook; and a nurse. When I am introduced to others, the first thing that they will know about me is that I am a nurse. Not because I will initially tell them, but the person who is introducing me will. How powerful is that? Our profession is so much a part of our identity. I think it stems from the innate respect that people have for us. That viewpoint comes with some responsibility and accountability. People view us as nurses twenty-four hours a day—not just during our work time. If we want to be viewed as professionals, we need to maintain a sense of professionalism beyond the work arena. Hmmm—maybe that is why we have vacations—so that we can leave town to be less restricted.

I will plan time to be myself in the midst of my professional obligations.

Notes

Notes

Notes

Notes

About the author

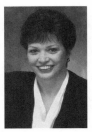

Gail Staudt, MSN, RN, CS, is a speaker, consultant, educator, author, and counselor in the field of health services. Gail has appeared on television, radio, international website interviews and conferences. Gail's thirty years in the nursing profession includes Critical Care nursing, nephrology nursing, forensic nursing, and holistic nursing. She has served as a nursing manager in several large healthcare facilities. Gail has been a member of the nursing faculty of the University of Pennsylvania, Jefferson University, Kutztown University, and St. Luke's Hospital School of Nursing. As a Psychiatric Advanced Practice Nurse, Gail has maintained a private therapy practice, with many clients in the healthcare field.

Gail holds a Nursing Diploma from Reading Hospital School of Nursing, a BSN magna cum laude from Kutztown University, an MSN magna cum laude from the University of Pennsylvania, and has completed post-graduate studies in Organizational Psychology at The Wharton School. She is listed in *Who's Who in American Nursing* and *Who's Who in Executive Women*. Gail is President and CEO of Gail Staudt & Associates, Inc. Visit with Gail at www.gail-staudt.com.